Table of Contents

Introduction..6

Chapter 1: What Is the Ketogenic Diet?......................8

The Benefits of Keto Diet..8

What to Eat on A Keto Diet?..10

Foods Not to Eat...10

Foods to Eat..11

Chapter 2: Your In-Depth Crockpot Guide for Delicious Dishes 13

The Benefits of Using a Crockpot.................................13

How Does It Work?...15

General Cooking Tips...16

Crockpot Safety Tips..18

Chapter 3: Chicken Keto Crockpot Recipes...................21

Lemon Grass and Coconut Chicken..........................21

Thai Chicken Soup...23

Keto Jerk Chicken..24

Three-Ingredient Crockpot Chicken Curry..............25

Crockpot Chicken with Bacon..................................26

Yellow Chicken Curry Soup.....................................27

Easy-Breezy Fajita Chicken.....................................29

Chicken Lemon Parsley Butter................................30

Chicken Heart Stroganoff..31

Lemony Rosemary Chicken.....................................33

Spicy Mexican Chicken Soup..................................35

Chocolate Chicken Mole Soup.................................37

Rosemary Turkey and Kale Soup............................ 39

Two-Ingredient Crockpot Chicken.........................40

Simple Slow Cooker Shredded Chicken.................. 41

Chapter 4: Beef and Lamb Keto Crockpot Recipes......................42

Lazy Man's Beef Stroganoff....................................42

Keto Crockpot Beef Stew...................................... 44

Crockpot Shredded Beef.. 46

Crockpot Taco Meat.. 47

Exotic Middle Eastern Beef...................................49

Slow Cooker Pot Roast..50

Tamil Attukal Paya Dish.. 51

Onion and Bison Soup... 53

Pepper Beef Tongue Stew......................................54

Mexican Beef Chili..56

Ground Beef Minestrone Soup.............................. 58

Slow Cooker Meatballs.. 60

Bacon, Chuck Roast and Cabbage Stew................. 61

Corned Beef Brisket with Cabbages...................... 62

Pot Roast Soup..63

Crockpot Ropa Vieja... 64

Indian Beef Stew...66

Clear Beef Shin Soup with Herbs.......................... 68

Crockpot Unspicy Beef Chili................................. 69

Island Lamb Stew.. 70

Chapter 5: Pork Keto Crockpot Recipes...................... 71

Pork Stew with Oyster Mushrooms........................ 71

Simple Three-Ingredient Pork Loin...................73

Easy Pork Luau...................74

Crockpot Pork Carnitas................... 76

Mexican Carne Adovada...................77

Spicy and Chili Pulled Pork...................79

Pulled Pork Cucumber Sliders...................81

Five-Spice Crockpot Pork Ribs...................83

Simple Pork Shanks Stew...................84

Creamy Coconut Curry Pork...................86

Balsamic Pork Tenderloin...................88

Pork Medallions in Mushroom Sauce................... 89

Pork Chops with Creamy Herbed Sauce................... 90

Jerk BBQ Pork Ribs...................92

Buffalo Pork Chops...................93

Chapter 6: Seafood Keto Crockpot Recipes................... 94

Spicy Shrimp Fra Diavolo................... 94

Savory and Spicy Garlicky Shrimp...................96

Shrimp Scampi with Spaghetti Squash................... 97

Tuna and White Beans...................98

Crockpot Swordfish Steaks................... 99

Rustic Fish and Tomatoes...................100

Sweet and Sour Shrimp................... 101

Lazyman's Seafood Stew................... 102

Halibut Vinaigrette...................104

Crockpot Crab Legs................... 105

Asian-Inspired Ginger Tuna Steaks...................106

Rustic Buttered Mussels..107

Boiled Lobster Tails.. 108

Creamy Shrimp Chowder.. 109

Keto-Approved Clam Chowder...111

Chapter 7: Breakfast and Eggs Keto Crockpot Recipes...............113

Mocha Chia Pudding...113

Rustic Fisherman's Eggs... 114

Easy-Peasy Breakfast Frittata...115

Sausage and Eggs Breakfast Casserole...................................116

Eggs Poached in Spicy Tomato Sauce (Shakshouka)........... 118

Pine Nut Breakfast Meatballs... 120

Breakfast Dijon Pork "Skillet"... 121

Gluten-Free Sausage-Crusted Quiche................................... 122

Overnight Breakfast Casserole.. 123

Sausage Breakfast Frittata... 124

Conclusion..125

Introduction

The ketogenic (keto) diet encourages people to consume low amounts of carbohydrates thus promoting the liver to produce ketones and use it as energy. The body undergoes the state of ketosis thus it is able to burn off fats faster so you lose weight and improve the stability of your insulin levels.

Under this particular diet, your main goal is to include mostly protein-rich foods in your diet. Protein is an essential key in this particular diet but you have to take note that too much of it can lower your ketone levels and too little may lead to muscle loss. Having said this, you need to consume between 0.6 grams and 0.8 grams of protein per pound of lean body mass.

Preparing your food is critical for the success of the keto diet and this is where crockpots come in. Crockpots are nifty kitchen appliances that allow you to cook your food longer at lower temperature settings. As a result, food becomes more tender yet the nutrition as well as the natural juices from the ingredients are retained within the pot. You can cook whatever keto recipes you want and make them with more nutritional value compared to when you cook them in ordinary pots.

With the keto diet, you are required to prepare mostly meat dishes thus preparation usually takes a lot of time. With slow cookers or crockpots, you will be able to prepare meals and they will be ready by the time you get back home. This prevents you from grabbing high-carb snacks to satisfy your hunger as food will always be ready for you to eat.

Chapter 1: What Is the Ketogenic Diet?

The principle of the keto diet is to consume foods low in carbohydrates. It is similar with other low-carb diets such as the Low Carb High Fat Diet and The Atkins Diet but the main difference is that the ketogenic diet encourages the consumption of adequate amounts of proteins – not too much and not too few. In turn, the body becomes a fat-burning machine as it is pushed to the state of ketosis.

Under the state of ketosis, the liver produces molecules called ketones, which are used to fuel the body in the absence of glucose. This state can only occur if you limit the amount of your carbs and moderate your consumption of proteins as excess of it can be converted to blood sugar.

Thus, when you opt for the keto diet, the entire body runs entirely on fat thus your insulin levels become low while fat metabolism shoots up. You can say that it mimics the effects and benefits of fasting without you going hungry.

The Benefits of Keto Diet

There are many benefits that you can get from following the keto diet. The benefit stems from the fact that the body is encouraged to release ketone bodies that improve the fat burning capabilities of the body. Below are the benefits of the keto diet.

- **Weight loss:** Once the body starts producing ketone bodies, the most evident benefit is weight loss. Once the insulin levels drop, the fat metabolism is triggered thus the body uses up fat molecules to sustain the energy needs of the body. The best thing about the keto diet is that you can lose weight without going hungry.

- **Reversal of Type 2 diabetes:** Since the insulin levels is reduced and kept in a stable level, the ketogenic diet is excellent to reverse Type 2 diabetes. If you follow this diet for a long time, you will be able to stabilize your insulin levels so that you can utilize your blood sugar effectively.

- **Better mental focus:** Ketosis leads to a steady flow of ketones to the brain thus it helps you avoid any big swings from consumption of sugar. As a result, you will experience better mental focus as well as improved concentration.

- **Better endurance:** The keto diet can increase your endurance. The thing is that as your body's stored supply of carbohydrates (glycogen) can only last for a few hours, fat stores can last for a few weeks. So if you are burning fat, you are likely to have more energy thus more endurance. It is crucial to take note that ketosis is part of our evolutionary advantage that allows our ancestors to survive even on famine.

- **Reduce epileptic seizures:** Before the keto diet was used for weight loss, it was first used in treating epileptic seizures in children. In fact, even modern science acknowledges the benefits of keto diet to epilepsy as patients are fed with low-carb diet to manage their seizures.

- **Other possible benefits:** Other possible benefits of keto diet are reducing acne and migraine. Studies also show that people who are at risk of getting cancer, Alzheimer's or Parkinson's diseases can benefit from the keto diet.

What to Eat on A Keto Diet?

Planning ahead your meals is the key to a successful keto diet. Having a diet plan is very important so that you can remain in ketosis for a long time. So, what are the types of foods that you can eat under the keto diet? The main idea about the keto diet is to keep your carb intake limited. Below are the types of foods that you should and should not eat.

Foods Not to Eat

Under the keto diet, there are certain foods that you need to strictly avoid. Below are the types of foods that you should not eat.

- **Sugar:** Any forms of sugar–natural or refined– should be avoided at all cost. These include agave, maple syrup, coconut sugar, dates, and basically all types of sweeteners.
- **Grains:** Grains should be avoided because they contain high amounts of carbohydrates that will be converted into glucose. These include corn, wheat, cereal, and rice.
- **Fruits:** Fruits may be good but not for the keto diet. Avoid starchy fruits like bananas, apples, and oranges. You can eat berries but in moderate amounts.
- **Tubers:** Tubers or root crops should be avoided and these include potato, yams, sweet potatoes, and jicama to name a few.

Foods to Eat

While you are discouraged to eat most of your favorite comfort foods, there are still many filling foods that you are allowed to eat under the keto diet as follows:

- **Meats:** Lean meats from fish, beef, lamb, and poultry should be eaten at appropriate amounts.

- **Vegetables:** Particularly vegetables that grow above the ground, they contain fewer amounts of starches that do not hinder the fat metabolism of the body. Examples of vegetables that can be eaten on the ketogenic diet include broccoli, cauliflower, broccoli, and many others. You can also eat green leafy vegetables as they don't contain starch at all.
- **Nuts and seeds:** Nuts and seeds are good sources of healthy fats. Eat toasted or raw walnuts, macadamias, pistachios, and sunflower seeds to name a few.
- **High fat dairy:** If you want to eat dairy products, make sure that they are high fat. These include hard cheeses, butter, high fat cream, and full cream milk.
- **Fats:** Adequate amounts of healthy fats can also be included in your diet such as coconut oil, avocado, salad dressings, and saturated fats.
- **Low calorie sweeteners:** Low calorie sweeteners like stevia and erythritol are low in carbs and does not affect the blood sugar levels.
- **Berries:** Berries are low in glycemic index so they don't affect the blood sugar as much as bananas and apples. Eat adequate amounts of berries in the keto diet as a good source of antioxidants and nutrients.

It is important to take note that your consumption should equate to the ratio of 70% fat, 25% protein, and 5% carbs. This means that you only need to consume at the most 30 grams of net carbs daily.

Chapter 2: Your In-Depth Crockpot Guide for Delicious Dishes

Crockpots are also called slow cookers. They are considered as a great time-saving kitchen device that is great for all types of cooks but most especially those who are novice in the kitchen. With this device, you can put every ingredient in the pot, turn it on and wait for it to cook hours later. This means that you can prepare dinner in the morning and expect it to be done and piping hot once you get back home in the evening.

Cooking with crockpots may be very easy but there are certain things that you need to know so that you can create delicious dishes out of this humble kitchen appliance. Thus, this chapter is dedicated to what you need to know about crockpots so that you can optimize its uses.

The Benefits of Using a Crockpot

Cooking with a slow cooker is one of the best ways to save time as well as prepare delicious and nutritious meals. With a slow cooker, you can put your ingredients in the pot and it cooks the entire day slowly so that it becomes ready by the time you get back. Aside from convenience, there are also other benefits of using a crockpot. Below are the benefits of using a crockpot.

- **Mess-free:** Cooking with a crockpot is mess-free. The thing is that there are no dishes or cups that you need to clean as you pot all ingredients in the pot and you are good to go. Clean up of the crockpot is also a breeze as you can wipe it with a clean kitchen towel. You can also line heat-proof plastic in the crockpot so that the interior of the pot remains clean.

- **It requires less electricity:** To cook your food, crockpots do not require large amount of electricity to be able to do its work. Since it does not use a lot of energy, it does not also heat up your entire kitchen space compared to when you use an oven.

- **Use cheaper cuts of meat:** The condensation that occurs in the crockpots serve as self-basting machines thus cheaper cuts of meat become tender if cooked in a slow cooker.

- **Cooks flavorful dishes:** And since you can use cheaper cuts of meat in a crockpot, it does not mean that your food will become less tasty. In fact, vegetables that are cooked in a crockpot absorbs the flavor of the spices and the stock.

- **Allows you to adjust the temperature:** Crockpots come with both high and low settings so you can adjust the temperature as well as the cooking time of your food. If you are at home and you want to sauté or simmer your food faster, the high setting is perfect but if you want to leave your food to cook by itself, you need to select the low setting.

How Does It Work?

What makes crockpots great is that they simplify the cooking process so that you can prepare meals even if you have limited cooking skills or if you are cooking your way through your busy schedule. But how does it work? The thing is that understanding how crockpots work is essential so that you will be able to cook delicious food no matter what.

The success of the crockpot in slow cooking your food relies on its design. Crockpots are basically electric pots that come with stoneware inserts. So unlike conventional stove top cooking, slow cookers can consistently cook food at low temperature for 12 hours. The stoneware inserts trap heat thus it can cook food for a long period of time.

As a general rule, crockpots cook food under low temperature setting of 190 °F or 87 °C, which is under the boiling point temperature. Under the high setting, food is cooked at 250 °F or 121 °C. However, there are other brands that offer other temperature ranges so you have to choose the ones that you are comfortable working with. But if you are in doubt, stick with this temperature setting.

Food is cooked in its own juices for a period of several hours thus the dish embodies the rich and natural flavors of the ingredients. Moreover, the use of low heat to cook food steadily brings out the flavor of food giving the final dish extra richness.

You cook food by layering different ingredients on the pot and cooking them for a few hours until they are done. The cooking time varies from one dish to another. As a general rule, side dishes as well as desserts can cook between 4 to 6 hours while meat dishes can take longer for about 6 to 10 hours. Some of the crockpots also feature a high temperature setting so that foods can be cooked between 3 and 4 hours.

General Cooking Tips

Just like other types of cooking appliances, there are some things that you need to know about crockpots so that you can cook delicious food even if it is your first time using it. Below are the general cooking tips that you need to know by heart when using your crockpot.

- **Cook just enough:** Fill the crockpot with ½ to ¾ full of ingredients including liquid. The thing is that your food will not cook through if it is full to the brim. On the other hand, if the food level is lower than recommended, it may lead to your food cooking quickly thus resulting to burning.

- **Place dry ingredients at the bottom:** The ingredients placed at the bottom of the crockpot cooks faster than those placed on top. Moreover, ingredients at the bottom also have more moisture than ingredients at the top because they are soaked in the simmering liquid. Thus said, place ingredients that are dry at the bottom of the crockpot.

- **Meat requires at least 8 hours of cooking:** Most meats from poultry to beef requires at least 8 hours of cooking. You can use different types of meat cuts and they will cook moist and tender after 8 hours.

- **Remove skin and fat from meats:** Whether you are cooking poultry or red meat, it is recommended that you remove skin and fat from meat. The thing is that fat melts if subjected to long cooking time thus it adds an unpleasant texture to the dish. Moreover, fats also cook the food quickly thus it may lead to having a dry texture if cooked for a long time in a slow cooker.

- **Always follow the layering instructions of ingredients:** While there is no specific layering instruction that you can follow, you need to cook the vegetables at the bottom while the meat should be on top where it is nearer the heating element.

- **Never lift the lid while cooking on low setting:** You don't need to stir your food if you are cooking in the low setting thus there is no need to lift the lid. The thing is that every time you lift the lid, heat will escape from the pot thus affecting the cooking time such that you need to extend to a few minutes to cook your food. Checking the progress of your food is easy as the crockpot comes with a glass lid. You just need to spin the cover without removing it from the pot to remove the condensation so that you can see your food inside the pot.

- **Use the high setting to thicken sauces:** If you are planning on adding thickeners, opt for the high setting during the last hour of the cooking time and add the cornstarch slurry. Stir the liquid to evenly thicken the sauce and wait for 15 minutes.

Crockpot Safety Tips

Slow cookers are designed to cook food for a few hours at a time by heating food properly at low temperature. Food is cooked at a low temperature which may lead bacterial colonies to populate your food. Thus, it is important that your food is fully cooked within 4 hours to avoid harboring bad bacteria. To avoid problems regarding the possible spoiling of food, below are crockpot safety tips that you need to be aware of and put into practice.

- **Ensure that the work area is clean:** Make sure that the work area around your crockpot is clean to avoid contamination of your food.

- **Prepare meat and veggies separately:** If you are preparing meat and vegetables beforehand, make sure that you prepare and store them separately to avoid cross-contamination.

- **Thaw the meat before putting in the slow cooker:** Defrost your meats so that they will cook all the way through the cooking duration. Moreover, it also allows the meat to achieve safe internal temperature thus preventing the risk of food poisoning.

- **Pay attention to the temperature:** It is crucial that the crockpot reaches a temperature that will effectively kill bacteria. You can start with the highest temperature setting for an hour and switch to low for the remaining cooking time. Although this may be the case, it is still safe to cook food at low temperature especially if you have to leave for work. Just use a food thermometer to check the internal temperature of your meat to see if it is cooked through.

- **Make sure that your food fits inside the pot:** Never fill the crockpot full to the brim. To effectively cook your food, the pot should be filled with ½ or ¾ full.

- **Cut up your meat:** Cut your meat up before putting them in the slow cooker so that they do not cook for a long time as well as they cook all the way through the meat.

Chapter 3: Chicken Keto Crockpot Recipes

Lemon Grass and Coconut Chicken

The lemon grass and coconut combination provides a creamy dish that is not only filling but also nutritious.

Yields: 6
Preparation Time: 20 minutes
Cooking Time: 5 hours

Ingredients:
- 10 chicken drumsticks, skin removed
- Salt and pepper to taste
- 1 stalk of lemon grass, trimmed
- 4 cloves of garlic, minced
- 1 piece ginger, sliced thinly
- 1 cup coconut milk
- 3 tablespoon coconut aminos
- 2 tablespoon fish sauce
- 1 teaspoon five spice powder
- 1 green onion, chopped

Instructions:
1) In a large bowl, season the chicken drumstick with salt and pepper.
2) Place the lemon grass, garlic, ginger, coconut milk, coconut aminos, fish sauce, and five spice powder in a blender or food processor. Blend until smooth.
3) Place the chicken in the slow cooker and pour over the marinade. Mix well.

4) Set the crockpot to low and cook for 4 to 5 hours.
5) Once done, serve with green onions.

Nutrition information: Calories per serving: 455; Carbohydrates: 5.38g; Protein: 40.89g; Fat: 29.57 g; Sugar: 2.65g; Sodium: 718mg; Fiber: 0.49 g

Thai Chicken Soup

This chicken recipe is a clear soup that is not only filling but also protein rich. It is a great dish for a cold rainy day.

Yields: 10
Preparation Time: 10 minutes
Cooking Time: 10 hours

Ingredients:
- 1 whole chicken, sliced into thick parts
- 1 stalk lemon grass, cut into large chunks
- 20 fresh basil leaves
- 1 thumb-size ginger, sliced thickly
- 1 tablespoon salt
- 3 cups water
- 1 lime, juice squeezed

Instructions:
1) Place all ingredients in the crockpot except the lime juice.
2) Cook on low for 8 to 10 hours.
3) Add lime juice once cooked.

Nutrition information: Calories per serving: 152; Carbohydrates: 0.44g; Protein: 27.7g; Fat: 3.69 g; Sugar: 0.08g; Sodium: 801mg; Fiber:0 g

Keto Jerk Chicken

This savory chicken dish can also be a perfect snack. It is salty, savory, and aromatic at the same time.

Yields: 4
Preparation Time: 10 minutes
Cooking Time: 5 hours

Ingredients:
- 4 teaspoons paprika
- 4 teaspoons salt
- 1 teaspoon cayenne pepper
- 2 teaspoons thyme
- 2 teaspoon onion powder
- 2 teaspoon garlic powder
- 1 teaspoon black pepper
- 5 chicken drumsticks, skin removed

Instructions:
1) Make a spice rub by combining in a bowl paprika, salt, cayenne pepper, thyme, onion powder, garlic powder and black pepper.
2) Coat the chicken with the spice rub and place inside the crockpot.
3) Set the temperature to low heat and cook for 6 hours or until the chicken meat falls off the bone.

Nutrition information: Calories per serving: 281; Carbohydrates: 4.31 g; Protein: 30.24 g; Fat: 15.38 g; Sugar: 0.41 g; Sodium: 2501 mg; Fiber: 1.5 g

Three-Ingredient Crockpot Chicken Curry

A creamy dish made only of three ingredients, this chicken curry recipe is very easy to make.

Yields: 8
Preparation Time: 10 minutes
Cooking Time: 5 hours

Ingredients:
- 3 pounds boneless chicken thighs, skin removed
- 3 tablespoon commercial green curry paste
- 1 can coconut milk

Instructions:
1) Place all ingredients in the crockpot.
2) Set the cooking time to low and cook for 5 hours.

Nutrition information: Calories per serving: 246; Carbohydrates: 1.32g; Protein: 47.29g; Fat: 4.58g; Sugar: 0.07g; Sodium: 180mg; Fiber: 1.3 g

Crockpot Chicken with Bacon

Who says that bacon and chicken are bad combination? This dish is a perfect pair for your vegetable salad.

Yields: 4
Preparation Time: 10 minutes
Cooking Time: 8 hours

Ingredients:
- 5 chicken breasts
- 10 slices of bacon
- 2 tablespoons thyme
- 1 tablespoon oregano
- 1 tablespoon rosemary
- 1 tablespoon salt

Instructions:
1) Place all ingredients in the crockpot and mix together to coat the chicken with the spices.
2) Set the crockpot to low and cook for 8 hours.
3) Once the chicken is cook, shred the meat.

Nutrition information: Calories per serving: 434; Carbohydrates: 0.92g; Protein: 83.81g; Fat: 59.1g; Sugar: 0.54g; Sodium: 2278mg; Fiber: 0.2 g

Yellow Chicken Curry Soup

This creamy chicken curry soup is not only flavorful but also spicy. Thanks to its spicy taste, it will surely amp your metabolism to burn more fats.

Yields: 2
Preparation Time: 10 minutes
Cooking Time: 6 hours

Ingredients:
- 1 cup onion, chopped
- 1 cup broccoli, chopped
- 1 cup tomatoes
- ½-pound of boneless chicken breast, skin removed
- 1 can coconut milk
- 1 tablespoon cumin
- 1 teaspoon ginger, minced
- 1 teaspoon coriander, ground
- 2 teaspoons garlic powder
- ½ teaspoon cayenne pepper
- 1 teaspoon cinnamon
- 1 cup water
- Salt to taste

Instructions:
1) Place the onion, broccoli, and tomatoes at the bottom of the crockpot. Add the chicken on top.
2) In a bowl, mix together coconut milk, cumin, ginger, coriander, garlic powder, cayenne pepper and cinnamon.
3) Pour over the chicken.

4) Add in the water and season with salt.
5) Cook at low temperature setting for 6 hours.

Nutrition information: Calories per serving: 204; Carbohydrates: 13.91g; Protein: 28.61 g; Fat:4.07 g; Sugar: 4.71 g; Sodium: 73 mg; Fiber: 3.8 g

Easy-Breezy Fajita Chicken

This fajita dish is very easy to make and it removes the hassle of preparation as all you need to do is to dump all ingredients in the pot.

Yields: 8
Preparation Time: 10 minutes
Cooking Time: 6 hours

Ingredients:
- 2 pounds boneless chicken breast, skin removed
- 1 small onion, sliced thinly
- 4 cloves of garlic, minced
- 2 cups bell pepper, sliced
- 1 can diced tomatoes
- 1 teaspoon salt
- 1 teaspoon oregano
- 1 teaspoon coriander, ground
- ½ teaspoon cumin
- ½ teaspoon chili powder

Instructions:
1) Place the chicken at the bottom of the crockpot and add the onions, garlic and bell peppers.
2) Pour over the diced tomatoes.
3) Stir in the rest of the ingredients.
4) Cook at low temperature setting for 6 hours.

Nutrition information: Calories per serving: 151; Carbohydrates: 3.44 g; Protein: 26.18 g; Fat: 3.13 g; Sugar: 1.59 g; Sodium: 376 mg; Fiber: 0.9 g

Chicken Lemon Parsley Butter

A delectable chicken dish that is made more refreshing with lemon, parsley and butter.

Yields: 8
Preparation Time: 10 minutes
Cooking Time: 8 hours

Ingredients:
- 1 whole roasting chicken
- Salt and pepper to taste
- 1 cup water
- 4 tablespoons butter
- 2 tablespoon fresh parsley, chopped
- 1 whole lemon, thinly sliced

Instructions:
1) Pat dry the chicken and rub with salt and pepper.
2) Place it at the middle of the crockpot and pour over water.
3) Cook on low for 6 to 8 hours or high for 3 hours.
4) Check if the internal temperature of the bird is 165 ºF to ensure that it is done.
5) Slather the chicken with butter and sprinkle parsley and slices of lemon on top.

Nutrition information: Calories per serving: 300; Carbohydrates: g; Protein: 29g; Fat: 18g; Sugar: 0.3g; Sodium: 175mg; Fiber: 0.1g

Chicken Heart Stroganoff

This stroganoff recipe might be made from chicken hearts but they are as delicious as beef.

Yields: 8
Preparation Time: 20 minutes
Cooking Time: 8 hours

Ingredients:
- 1 pound whole mushroom, sliced
- 1 onion, sliced thinly
- 2 pounds chicken hearts, cut lengthwise
- 4 cloves of garlic, minced
- ½ tablespoon paprika
- 1 tablespoon Dijon mustard
- ½ tablespoon cayenne pepper
- Salt and pepper to taste
- 1 cup chicken stock
- ¼ cup coconut cream
- 7 ounces commercial Greek yogurt, plain

Instructions:
1) Place the mushrooms and onions at the bottom of the crockpot.
2) Add the chicken hearts on top.
3) Add the garlic, paprika, mustard, and cayenne pepper. Season with salt and pepper.
4) Pour in the chicken stock.
5) Cook for 6 to 8 hours.
6) Once done, stir in the coconut cream and yogurt.
7) Cook on high for 10 minutes before serving.

Nutrition information: Calories per serving: 385; Carbohydrates: 12.98g; Protein: 25.35g; Fat: 14g; Sugar: 3.33g; Sodium: 182mg; Fiber: 7g

Lemony Rosemary Chicken

A light and savory chicken crockpot dish that is perfect for all occasions.

Yields: 6
Preparation Time: 20 minutes
Cooking Time: 6 hours

Ingredients:
- 1 tablespoon olive oil
- 3 onions, sliced
- 6 cloves garlic, chopped
- 4 pounds chicken thighs, skin removed
- Salt and pepper to taste
- 3 sprigs of rosemary
- ½ cup lemon juice
- ¾ cup chicken broth
- 1 tablespoon lemon zest
- 1 lemon sliced thinly for garnish

Instructions:
1) Heat the crockpot to high and pour in oil. Sauté the onions and garlic until slightly browned.
2) Add the chicken and season with salt and pepper to taste.
3) Stir in the rest of the ingredients except the lemon slices.
4) Cook for 6 hours.
5) Garnish with lemon slices.

Nutrition information: Calories per serving: 706; Carbohydrates: 5.15 g; Protein: 50.65g; Fat: 52.65g; Sugar: 1.52 g; Sodium: 362 mg; Fiber: 0.3 g

Spicy Mexican Chicken Soup

This chicken soup has some kick to it. It is a great dish to boost your body's metabolism.

Yields: 8
Preparation Time: 10 minutes
Cooking Time: 6 to 8 hours

Ingredients:
- 1 cup onions, diced
- 4 teaspoon minced garlic
- ½ cup roma tomatoes
- ¼ cup jalapeno, seeds removed
- 4 cups chicken breast, skin removed
- 1 ¾ cup tomato juice
- 6 cups chicken broth
- 1 teaspoon coriander, ground
- 1 tablespoon cumin, ground
- 1 tablespoon chili powder
- Salt to taste
- 2 tablespoon lime juice
- Cilantro for garnish

Instructions:
1) Place the onion, garlic, tomatoes, and jalapeno at the bottom of the crockpot.
2) Add the chicken on top.
3) Pour in the tomato juice and chicken broth.
4) Stir in coriander, cumin, and chili powder. Season with salt.
5) Cook for 6 to 8 hours.

6) Garnish with lime juice and cilantro.

Nutrition information: Calories per serving: 286; Carbohydrates: 6.14g; Protein: 32.48g; Fat: 14.3 g; Sugar: 3.28 g; Sodium: 876mg; Fiber: 1.9g

Chocolate Chicken Mole Soup

This classic Mexican dish is not only rich in protein but also in taste.

Yields: 6
Preparation Time: 15 minutes
Cooking Time: 6 hours

Ingredients:
- 2 pounds chicken breast, skin removed
- salt and pepper to taste
- 2 tablespoons butter
- 1 onion, chopped
- 4 cloves of garlic, crushed
- 7 tomatoes, chopped
- 5 Mexican chili peppers, chopped
- ¼ cup almond butter
- ½ teaspoon chili powder
- Avocado and cilantro for garnish

Instructions:
1) In a bowl, season chicken with salt and pepper.
2) Set the crockpot to high and melt the butter. Sauté the onions and garlic for three minutes until slightly brown.
3) Add the tomatoes, chili peppers, and chicken.
4) Add the almond butter and chili powder.
5) Set to low temperature and cook for 6 hours.
6) Garnish with avocado slices and cilantro.

Nutrition information: Calories per serving: 451; Carbohydrates: 13.6 g; Protein: 36.19g; Fat: 28.9 g; Sugar: 5.58g; Sodium: 167mg; Fiber: 5.6 g

Rosemary Turkey and Kale Soup

This aromatic turkey soup is made more nutritious with superfood kale.

Yields: 6
Preparation Time: 10 minutes
Cooking Time: 8 hours

Ingredients:
- ½ tablespoon butter
- ½ of onion, chopped
- 2 cloves garlic, minced
- 3 cups turkey meat, chopped into chunks
- salt and pepper to taste
- 4 cups chicken stock
- 2 sprigs of rosemary
- 3 cups kale, chopped

Instructions:
1) Set the crockpot to high heat and melt the butter. Add the onions and garlic for three minutes or until slightly browned.
2) Add the turkey meat and season with salt and pepper.
3) Stir in the rest of the ingredients.
4) Cook on low temperature for 8 hours.

Nutrition information: Calories per serving: 204; Carbohydrates: 5.79g; Protein: 21.03g; Fat: 7.68g; Sugar: 5.5g; Sodium: 650mg; Fiber: 1g

Two-Ingredient Crockpot Chicken

This crockpot chicken dish is very easy to make and all it takes are two ingredients to create a world-class dish.

Yields: 4
Preparation Time: 10 minutes
Cooking Time: 5 hours

Ingredients:
- 3 pounds chicken breast
- 1 ounce of commercial salsa verde

Instructions:
1) Place all ingredients in the crockpot.
2) Stir in to mix everything.
3) Set the temperature to low and cook for 5 hours.
4) Once cooked, shred the meat with fork.

Nutrition information: Calories per serving: 588; Carbohydrates: 0.45 g; Protein: 71.01g; Fat: 31.35g; Sugar: 0.25 g; Sodium: 257mg; Fiber: 0.1g

Simple Slow Cooker Shredded Chicken

This savory shredded chicken is very delectable but does not require a lot of kitchen labor.

Yields: 12
Preparation Time: 10 minutes
Cooking Time: 8 hours

Ingredients:
- 6 pounds chicken breast, skin removed
- 1 teaspoon salt
- ½ teaspoon pepper
- 5 cups chicken broth
- 2 tablespoons butter

Instructions:
1) Place the chicken in the middle of the crockpot and season with salt and pepper.
2) Add the broth.
3) Cook for 8 hours.
4) Once cooked, shred the chicken with fork and add the butter and allow it to melt.

Nutrition information: Calories per serving: 414; Carbohydrates: 0.64g; Protein: 48 g; Fat: 23.12 g; Sugar: 0.54g; Sodium: 737mg; Fiber: 0g

Chapter 4: Beef and Lamb Keto Crockpot Recipes

Lazy Man's Beef Stroganoff

Traditional beef stroganoff is very difficult to prepare but with a slow cooker, it is as easy as 1-2-3.

Yields: 6
Preparation Time: 15 minutes
Cooking Time: 5 hours

Ingredients:
- 1 teaspoon garlic powder
- 2 teaspoons paprika
- 1 teaspoon thyme
- 1 teaspoon onion powder
- 2 pounds beef meat, any cut
- 2 teaspoons salt
- ½ teaspoon pepper
- 8 ounces mushroom, sliced
- ½ onion, sliced
- 1/3 cup coconut cream
- 2 teaspoon red wine vinegar

Instructions:
1) In a small bowl, mix together garlic powder, paprika, thyme, and onion powder. Set aside.
2) Season beef with salt and pepper. Add in the dry spice rub.
3) Place the mushrooms and onions in the crockpot.

4) Add the seasoned beef.
5) Cook for 5 hours.
6) During the last hour, pour over the coconut cream and red wine vinegar.

Nutrition information: Calories per serving: 533; Carbohydrates: 7.8g; Protein: 36.44g; Fat: 27.06g; Sugar: 1.18g; Sodium: 893mg; Fiber: 4.8g

Keto Crockpot Beef Stew

This dish is basically dump and cook so you don't need to spend a lot of time in the kitchen to enjoy this hearty dish.

Yields: 12
Preparation Time: 20 minutes
Cooking Time: 6 hours

Ingredients:
- 1 pound grass-fed beef, cubed
- 1 onion, chopped
- 1 zucchini, diced
- ½ can tomato paste
- 2 cloves of garlic, minced
- 2 sprigs of thyme
- 2 bay leaves
- 3 celery stalks
- 2 tablespoons parsley, chopped
- 2 tablespoon apple cider vinegar
- 3 cups green beans
- salt and pepper to taste
- 3 cups water

Instructions:
1) Place all ingredients in the crockpot.
2) Cook for 6 hours on low temperature.
3) Serve warm.

Nutrition information: Calories per serving: 95; Carbohydrates: 4.85g; Protein: 8.36g; Fat: 5.06 g; Sugar: 2.06g; Sodium: 36mg; Fiber: 1.3g

Crockpot Shredded Beef

You don't have to spend a lot of time slaving in the kitchen to make this shredded beef recipe but it is as delicious as traditional shredded beef recipes.

Yields: 5
Preparation Time: 5 minutes
Cooking Time: 8 hours

Ingredients:
- ¼ cup stock
- 4 pounds beef chuck roast
- salt and pepper to taste
- ½ teaspoon cumin
- ¼ teaspoon chili
- ½ tablespoon oregano
- ¼ teaspoon paprika
- 1/8 teaspoon cinnamon
- ½ teaspoon garlic powder
- 2 tablespoon tomato paste
- 2 cups water

Instructions:
1) Place all ingredients in the crockpot.
2) Cook for 8 hours on low heat.
3) Once cooked, shred the beef with two forks.
4) Serve with the juices of the beef roast.

Nutrition information: Calories per serving: 339; Carbohydrates: 1.29g; Protein: 48.78g; Fat:15.46g; Sugar: 0.64g; Sodium: 160mg; Fiber: 0.3g

Crockpot Taco Meat

Who doesn't love taco meat? But if you don't have enough time to make taco meat, you can always make taco meat using your crockpot.

Yields: 6
Preparation Time: 10 minutes
Cooking Time: 5 hours

Ingredients:
- 1 tablespoon chili powder
- ½ teaspoon coriander, ground
- 1 teaspoon cumin
- ½ teaspoon dried oregano
- ½ teaspoon garlic powder
- ¼ teaspoon paprika
- ½ teaspoon onion powder
- ¼ teaspoon crushed red pepper
- 2 pounds ground beef
- 1 teaspoon salt
- 1 teaspoon black pepper
- 3 tablespoon tomato paste

Instructions:
1) In a mixing bowl, mix together the chili powder, coriander, cumin, oregano, garlic powder, paprika, onion powder, and crushed red pepper. Set aside.
2) Season the ground beef with salt and pepper to taste.
3) Rub the ground beef with the spice rub and place it in the crockpot.
4) Add the tomato paste.

5) Cook on low for 5 hours.
6) Once cooked, break up the meat with a slotted spoon.

Nutrition information: Calories per serving: 399; Carbohydrates: 3.11g; Protein:38.9g; Fat: 24.8g; Sugar: 1.12g; Sodium: 533mg; Fiber:1.1 g

Exotic Middle Eastern Beef

This dish might be exotic but it is very easy to make and you don't have to struggle in the kitchen to make this dish.

Yields: 8
Preparation Time: 20 minutes
Cooking Time: 8 hours

Ingredients:
- 3 pounds beef brisket
- Salt and pepper to taste
- 1 teaspoon fennel seeds
- 1 teaspoon whole cloves
- ½ teaspoon whole peppercorns
- 1 teaspoon cumin powder
- 1 teaspoon cardamom powder
- ½ teaspoon ground cinnamon
- 3 tablespoon tomato paste
- ½ onion, chopped
- 3 cups bone broth
- ¼ cup coconut vinegar

Instructions:
1) Place all ingredients in the pot.
2) Cook at low temperature for 8 hours.
3) Once cooked, shred with fork.

Nutrition information: Calories per serving: 563; Carbohydrates: 5.14g; Protein: 40.91g; Fat: 40.86g; Sugar: 2.23g; Sodium: 3321mg; Fiber: 1.2g

Slow Cooker Pot Roast

It is difficult to make your own pot roast with this crockpot recipe. You can just dump the ingredients in the crockpot and it will be ready by the time you are home.

Yields: 6
Preparation Time: 10 minutes
Cooking Time: 10 hours

Ingredients:
- 2 pounds beef arm or chuck roast, trimmed from fat and patted dry
- 1 ½ teaspoon salt
- ¾ teaspoon black pepper
- 2 tablespoons basil, chopped
- ½ cup onion, chopped
- 4 cloves of garlic, minced
- 2 bay leaves
- 2 cup beef stock

Instructions:
1) Place all ingredients in the crockpot.
2) Close the lid and cook on low for 10 hours.
3) Remove the bay leaves.
4) Serve with the thickened sauce.

Nutrition information: Calories per serving: 234; Carbohydrates: 2.4g; Protein: 33.1g; Fat: 10.3g; Sugar: 1g; Sodium: 101.3mg; Fiber: 0.1g

Tamil Attukal Paya Dish

Attukal Paya or Lamb's Feet Soup is a traditional Southern Indian dish. Recreate this traditional spicy Indian food with your crockpot.

Yields: 10
Preparation Time: 10 minutes
Cooking Time: 10 hours

Ingredients:
- 1 ½ pounds lamb fee, cut into chunks
- 1 onion, chopped
- 3 cloves of garlic
- 1 teaspoon black peppercorns
- 1-inch ginger, sliced thinly
- 1 can tomatoes
- 1 teaspoon coriander, ground
- ½ teaspoon cayenne pepper powder
- 1 bay leaf
- 4 cups water

Instructions:
1) Broil the lamb fee first in the oven for 10 minutes to add a roasted flavor on the soup.
2) Meanwhile, mix all other ingredients except the bay leaf and water in a food processor and pulse until fine.
3) Place the lamb feet in the crockpot and pour over the sauce.
4) Add the bay leaf and water.
5) Cook on low for 10 hours.

Nutrition information: Calories per serving: 184; Carbohydrates: 2.27g; Protein: 17.06g; Fat: 11.51g; Sugar: 1.1g; Sodium: 76 mg; Fiber: 0.6g

Onion and Bison Soup

This savory onion and bison soup is one hearty recipe that will surely warm your heart and stomach.

Yields: 8
Preparation Time: 10 minutes
Cooking Time: 6 hours

Ingredients:
- 1 tablespoon olive oil
- 6 onions, sliced
- 2 pounds bison roast
- 4 cups beef stock
- ½ cup sherry
- 3 sprigs of thyme
- 1 bay leaf
- salt and pepper to taste

Instructions:
1) Set the cooking on high and add the olive oil. Sauté the onions until brown.
2) Add the rest of the ingredients and close the lid.
3) Set the cooking time on low and cook for 6 hours

Nutrition information: Calories per serving: 212; Carbohydrates: 4.3g; Protein: 25.78g; Fat: 10.34g; Sugar: 1.47g; Sodium: 342mg; Fiber: 0.3 g

Pepper Beef Tongue Stew

People don't really like to eat offal but this beef tongue stew does not even taste like one.

Yields: 10
Preparation Time: 15 minutes
Cooking Time: 8 hours

Ingredients:
- 3 pounds sliced beef tongue, boiled and cleaned
- 1 onion, chopped
- 6 cloves of garlic, minced
- 1 red bell pepper, diced
- 1 yellow bell pepper, diced
- 2 cups chicken stock
- 8-ounce can of tomato sauce
- 2 jalapeno peppers, diced
- salt and pepper to taste
- 1 teaspoon Cajun spice
- 1 ¾ stick of butter
- 1 bunch of green onion, chopped

Instructions:
1) Place the beef tongue, onion, garlic, and bell peppers in the crockpot.
2) Add the chicken stock and tomato sauce. Stir in the jalapeno pepper and season with salt, pepper and Cajun spice.
3) Cook on low temperature for 8 hours.
4) Once cooked, add butter and garnish with green onions.

Nutrition information: Calories per serving: 441; Carbohydrates: 9.39g; Protein: 28.57g; Fat: 31.07g; Sugar: 4.45g; Sodium: 462mg; Fiber: 1.9g

Mexican Beef Chili

Get a boost in your metabolism with this spicy beef chili recipe. It is a delicious one-pot dish that anyone can make.

Yields: 8
Preparation Time: 10 minutes
Cooking Time: 8 hours

Ingredients:
- 1 onion, chopped
- 2 cloves of garlic, minced
- 4 stalks of celery, chopped
- 2-pound ground beef
- 8 ounces of canned tomatoes
- 1 cup fresh tomatoes, diced
- 2 tablespoon chili powder
- 1 tablespoon cumin
- 2 teaspoons smoked paprika
- salt and pepper to taste
- a dash of smoked paprika

Instructions:
1) Place the onions, garlic and celery at the bottom of the crockpot.
2) Add the ground beef and make sure that the meat is crumbled.
3) Pour in the canned tomatoes and fresh tomatoes.
4) Add the rest of the spices and seasonings.
5) Cook on low for 8 hours or on high for 6 hours.

Nutrition information: Calories per serving: 316; Carbohydrates: 5.66g; Protein: 29.88g; Fat: 19.01g; Sugar: 2.42g; Sodium: 176mg; Fiber: 2.2g

Ground Beef Minestrone Soup

This simple minestrone soup is not only heart-warming but also very nutritious. It is a complete meal that will satisfy your stomach.

Yields: 8
Preparation Time: 10 minutes
Cooking Time: 8 hours

Ingredients:
- 1 pound ground beef
- 1 onion, diced
- 1 tablespoon garlic, minced
- 3 cups of water
- 2 small zucchinis, diced
- 1 stalk celery, diced
- ½ cup vegetable broth
- 1 can diced tomatoes
- ½ teaspoon basil
- ½ teaspoon dried oregano

Instructions:
1) Set the crockpot on high and add the ground beef. Stir in the onion and garlic and sauté for 3 minutes or until meat is slightly browned.
2) Add water and the rest of the ingredients.
3) Adjust the temperature and cook on low for 8 hours.

Nutrition information: Calories per serving: 157; Carbohydrates: 2.86g; Protein: 14.38g; Fat:9.27g; Sugar:1.36g; Sodium: 104mg; Fiber: 0.8g

Slow Cooker Meatballs

This crockpot meatball recipe is great by itself or with zucchini noodles.

Yields: 8
Preparation Time: 20 minutes
Cooking Time: 5 hours

Ingredients:
- 3 pounds ground beef
- ¼ cup spinach, finely chopped
- 2 tablespoons onion, chopped
- 1 teaspoon garlic powder
- salt and pepper to taste
- 1 can commercial pasta sauce

Instructions:
1) In a mixing bowl, mix together the beef, spinach, onion, and garlic powder.
2) Season with salt and pepper.
3) Using your hands, form small meatballs and place them carefully in the crockpot.
4) Add the commercial pasta sauce. Be careful not to damage the meatballs.
5) Cook on low for 5 hours.

Nutrition information: Calories per serving: 437; Carbohydrates: 1.08g; Protein: 43.18g; Fat: 27.53g; Sugar: 0.41g; Sodium: 115mg; Fiber: 0.2g

Bacon, Chuck Roast and Cabbage Stew

A simple comfort food recipe, this chuck roast recipe is a hearty dish that will satisfy not only your hunger but also your soul.

Yields: 8
Preparation Time: 10 minutes
Cooking Time: 7 hours

Ingredients:
- ½ pound uncured bacon strips
- 2 onions, sliced
- 1 clove of garlic, crushed
- 3 pounds chuck roast cut into 2-inch thick pieces
- 1 small cabbage, sliced
- 1 sprig of thyme
- 1 cup beef bone broth
- salt and pepper to taste

Instructions:
1) Place the bacon slices in the bottom of the crockpot.
2) Add the onion and garlic.
3) Pour in the chuck roast on top followed by the cabbage slices.
4) Add the thyme and broth.
5) Season with salt and pepper.
6) Cook on low for 7 hours.

Nutrition information: Calories per serving: 309; Carbohydrates: 8.9g; Protein: 35.88g; Fat: 14.77g; Sugar: 3.59g; Sodium: 1886mg; Fiber: 2.4g

Corned Beef Brisket with Cabbages

Corned beef is a great dish that you can eat all throughout the day. Add more nutritional value to this recipe by adding sliced cabbages.

Yields: 8
Preparation Time: 10 minutes
Cooking Time: 8 hours

Ingredients:
- 1 head cabbage, sliced
- ½ onion, sliced
- 1 stalk of celery, chopped
- 2 ½ pounds corned beef brisket
- 1 cup chicken stock

Instructions:
1) Place the cabbages and onions at the bottom of the crockpot.
2) Add in the celery and the corned beef brisket.
3) Pour in the chicken stock.
4) Cook on low for 8 hours.

Nutrition information: Calories per serving: 314; Carbohydrates: 6.6g; Protein: 22.6g; Fat: 21.6g; Sugar: 3.24g; Sodium: 1789mg; Fiber: 1.5g

Pot Roast Soup

Turn your pot roasts into this delicious soup recipe. Enjoy this hearty dish on a rainy day or cold night.

Yields: 4
Preparation Time: 15 minutes
Cooking Time: 8 hours

Ingredients:
- 1 ¼ pounds of meat stew
- 1 onion, diced
- 1 head cauliflower, diced
- 1 can diced tomatoes
- 1 Portobello mushroom, diced
- ¾ cup chicken stock
- 1 teaspoon dried basil
- 1 teaspoon dried oregano
- salt and pepper to taste

Instructions:
1) Add all ingredients in the crockpot.
2) Close the lid and cook on low for 8 hours or high for 5 hours.

Nutrition information: Calories per serving: 211; Carbohydrates: 5.21g; Protein: 21.63 g; Fat: 11.29g; Sugar: 2.47 g; Sodium: 138mg; Fiber: 1.5g

Crockpot Ropa Vieja

Ropa vieja is a Cuban shredded meat dish. Make this exotic dish with your crockpot.

Yields: 8
Preparation Time: 20 minutes
Cooking Time: 8 hours

Ingredients:
- 2 tablespoon coconut oil
- 3 pounds flank steak
- 2 cloves of garlic, minced
- 3 peppers, sliced
- ¼ cup parsley, chopped
- ¼ cup cilantro, chopped
- 1 cup water
- 1 tablespoon white wine vinegar
- 2 cans of tomato sauce
- 1 tablespoon onion powder
- 1 tablespoon cumin powder
- 1 tablespoon oregano
- salt to taste

Instructions:
1) In a skillet, heat oil and sear the flank steak for 3 minutes on each side. Set aside.
2) Place garlic, peppers, parsley, and cilantro in the crockpot.
3) Add in the seared flank steak.
4) Pour in water, vinegar, and tomato sauce.
5) Add in the onion powder, cumin and oregano.

6) Season with salt to taste.
7) Close the lid and cook on low for 8 hours.

Nutrition information: Calories per serving: 277; Carbohydrates: 3.01g; Protein: 37.13g; Fat: 12.14g; Sugar: 0.97g; Sodium: 95mg; Fiber: 0.6g

Indian Beef Stew

Recreate this Indian beef stew recipe in your crockpot. The best thing about this recipe is that you don't need to slave in your kitchen the entire day and it will come out as delicious as the traditional recipe.

Yields: 8
Preparation Time: 20 minutes
Cooking Time: 8 hours

Ingredients:
- ½ tablespoon oil
- 2 ½ pounds beef chunks
- 1 onion, diced
- 1 can tomatoes
- 2 cups beef stock
- 2 teaspoon ginger paste
- 2 teaspoon garlic, minced
- 2 tablespoon curry powder
- 2 teaspoon garam masala powder
- ¼ teaspoon ground cloves
- 2 bay leaves
- ¼ cup whipping cream
- ½ cup Greek yogurt

Instructions:
1) In a skillet, heat oil and sear the beef chunks. Set aside.
2) Place all ingredients in the crockpot except the whipping cream and yogurt.
3) Add the seared beef chunks.

4) Close the lid and cook on low for 8 hours.
5) Add the cream and yogurt before serving.

Nutrition information: Calories per serving: 134; Carbohydrates: 3.48g; Protein: 15.96g; Fat: 4.88g; Sugar: 2.91 g; Sodium: 183mg; Fiber: 1.8g

Clear Beef Shin Soup with Herbs

This clear beef soup is made more refreshing and aromatic with the herbs used. It will truly satisfy your hungry stomach.

Yields: 8
Preparation Time: 10 minutes
Cooking Time: 8 hours

Ingredients:
- 2 pounds beef shin, cut into chunks
- 1 onion, chopped
- 3 stalks of celery, chopped
- 2 cups beef stock
- 1 teaspoon cumin
- 1 teaspoon thyme
- 1 bay leaf
- 1 teaspoon parsley
- salt and pepper to taste

Instructions:
1) Place all ingredients in the crockpot.
2) Close the lid and cook on low for 8 hours.
3) Remove the bay leaf before serving.

Nutrition information: Calories per serving: 147; Carbohydrates: 2.88g; Protein: 25.88g; Fat: 3.69g; Sugar: 1.29g; Sodium: 197mg; Fiber: 0.5g

Crockpot Unspicy Beef Chili

Do you love to eat beef chili but don't like its spicy taste? This unspicy beef chili is the best recipe to follow.

Yields: 8
Preparation Time: 20 minutes
Cooking Time: 8 hours

Ingredients:
- 2 cans diced tomatoes
- 2 tablespoons smoked paprika
- 1 pound ground beef
- 1 onion, chopped
- 1 green bell pepper, chopped
- 8 ounces of Portobello mushrooms, sliced
- 2 cloves of garlic, minced
- 1 tablespoon butter
- salt and pepper to taste

Instructions:
1) Turn on the crockpot and set to high cooking setting.
2) Add the tomatoes and paprika and stir.
3) Stir in the ground beef and sauté for 3 minutes.
4) Add the rest of the ingredients.
5) Change the heat setting to low and cook for 8 hours.

Nutrition information: Calories per serving: 188; Carbohydrates: 6.42g; Protein: 16.3g; Fat: 11.15g; Sugar: 3.19g; Sodium: 110mg; Fiber: 2.5 g

Island Lamb Stew

This lamb recipe is very easy to make and all there is to it is to dump and forget everything until dinner time.

Yields: 4
Preparation Time: 15 minutes
Cooking Time: 8 hours

Ingredients:
- 1 tablespoon butter
- 1 cup onion, sliced
- 1 pound lamb, diced
- 1 cup celery, sliced
- ¾ cup green pepper, chopped
- 1 tablespoon curry powder
- 1 can tomatoes
- salt and pepper to taste

Instructions:
1) Set the crockpot to high heat and add butter.
2) Sauté the onions for a minute then add the lamb.
3) Sear the lamb for 3 minutes.
4) Pour the remaining ingredients.
5) Close the lid and set the heat to low.
6) Cook for 8 hours.

Nutrition information: Calories per serving: 352; Carbohydrates: 7.83g; Protein: 29.32g; Fat: 22.4 g; Sugar: 3.82g; Sodium: 187mg; Fiber: 2.9 g

Chapter 5: Pork Keto Crockpot Recipes

Pork Stew with Oyster Mushrooms

Pork is made refreshing with oyster mushrooms. This recipe is not only light but also very nutritious.

Yields: 4
Preparation Time: 15 minutes
Cooking Time: 6 hours

Ingredients:
- 2 tablespoon coconut oil
- 1 onion, chopped
- 1 clove of garlic, chopped
- 2 pounds pork loin
- salt and pepper to taste
- 2 tablespoon dried mustard
- 2 tablespoon dried oregano
- ½ teaspoon nutmeg powder
- 1 ½ cups bone broth
- 2 tablespoon white wine vinegar
- 2 pounds oyster mushroom
- ¼ cup coconut milk
- 3 tablespoon capers

Instructions:
1) Heat the crockpot to high and add coconut oil.

2) Sauté the onion and garlic for two minutes and add in the pork loin. Sear and season with salt and pepper to taste.
3) Stir in the mustard, oregano, and nutmeg.
4) Pour in the bone broth and white wine vinegar.
5) Add in the mushrooms.
6) Close the lid and adjust the cooking temperature to low.
7) Cook for 6 hours.
8) Ten minutes before the cooking time, add in the coconut milk and capers.

Nutrition information: Calories per serving: 734; Carbohydrates: 23.5g; Protein: 50.4g; Fat: 48.9g; Sugar: 4.3g; Sodium: 1118mg; Fiber: 7.9g

Simple Three-Ingredient Pork Loin

This pork loin recipe only requires three ingredients. And cooking it in a crockpot makes it easier!

Yields: 8
Preparation Time: 10 minutes
Cooking Time: 12 hours

Ingredients:
- 2 pounds pork loin
- 2 onions, chopped
- 3 cups beef stock

Instructions:
1) Place everything in the crockpot.
2) Cover the crockpot and set the cooking time to low.
3) Cook for 12 hours until the meat is tender and falls apart.

Nutrition information: Calories per serving: 260; Carbohydrates: 3.65g; Protein: 31.12g; Fat: 12.65g; Sugar: 1.65g; Sodium: 242mg; Fiber: 0.5 g

Easy Pork Luau

This Hawaiian dish is made easier with a crockpot. Simply dump the ingredients and you are good to go.

Yields: 10
Preparation Time: 15 minutes
Cooking Time: 7 hours

Ingredients:
- 4 slices of smoked bacon
- 5 cloves of garlic, minced
- 3 pounds pork roast shoulder
- 1 ½ tablespoon Hawaiian black lava sea salt or ordinary salt
- 2 tablespoon liquid smoke

Instructions:
1) Set the crockpot to high setting and place the raw bacon slices.
2) Sprinkle minced garlic over the bacon.
3) Using a knife, poke holes through the pork roast to allow heat and the sauce to seep into the meat.
4) Rub salt all over the pork. Place the pork inside the crockpot.
5) Add the liquid smoke.
6) Adjust the cooking setting and cook on low for 8 hours.
7) Shred the meat with fork.

Nutrition information: Calories per serving: 182; Carbohydrates: 2g; Protein: 14g; Fat: 13g; Sugar: 1g; Sodium: 1243mg; Fiber: 0.9g

Crockpot Pork Carnitas

This pork carnitas recipe is very easy and all there is to it is to dump everything and let it cook on its own while you do other more important things.

Yields: 10
Preparation Time: 10 minutes
Cooking Time: 6 hours

Ingredients:
- 2 ½ pounds boneless pork shoulder
- 5 cloves of garlic, minced
- 2 teaspoon ground cumin
- 2 teaspoons oregano
- 1 tablespoon sherry vinegar
- salt and pepper to taste
- 1 onion, quartered
- 4 bay leaves

Instructions:
1) Place pork, garlic, cumin, oregano, and sherry vinegar in the crockpot. Season with salt and pepper.
2) Add the onions and bay leaves.
3) Cover the crockpot and set on low temperature.
4) Cook for six hours.
5) Once done, shred the meat using fork.

Nutrition information: Calories per serving: 155; Carbohydrates: 2.29g; Protein: 25.96g; Fat: 3.99g; Sugar: 0.73g; Sodium: 63mg; Fiber: 0.4g

Mexican Carne Adovada

Whip up this exotic Mexican dish with your crockpot and be amazed of its flavors.

Yields: 12
Preparation Time: 8 hours
Cooking Time: 6 hours

Ingredients:
- 3 pounds pork shoulder, cut into cubes
- 8 ounces Mexican chilies
- 6 cloves of garlic, chopped
- 1 teaspoon cumin powder
- 2 teaspoons oregano
- 1 teaspoon coriander powder
- 2 cups beef stock
- 1 onion, chopped
- 2 teaspoon apple cider vinegar
- salt to taste

Instructions:
1) In a bowl, mix together, the pork shoulders, chilies, garlic, cumin, oregano and coriander. Let it rest for at least 8 hours to marinate.
2) Place the marinated meat in the crockpot and add beef stock, onions, and apple cider vinegar. Season with salt and pepper to taste.
3) Close the lid and set to low temperature.
4) Cook for 6 hours.
5) Serve with the thickened sauce.

Nutrition information: Calories per serving: 334; Carbohydrates: 3.11g; Protein: 31.67g; Fat: 20.79g; Sugar: 1.17g; Sodium: 209mg; Fiber: 0.4g

Spicy and Chili Pulled Pork

Add a little kick to your pulled pork recipe by making this spicy and chili pulled pork using your crockpot.

Yields: 8
Preparation Time: 10 minutes
Cooking Time: 10 hours

Ingredients:
- 2 pounds pork roast, trimmed from fat
- 3 cloves of garlic, minced
- 2 onions, diced
- 1 bell pepper, diced
- 1 can of tomato sauce
- 2 cans of roasted tomatoes
- 2 tablespoon garlic powder
- ½ cup hot sauce
- 3 tablespoons smoked paprika
- 1 teaspoon cumin
- 2 tablespoon chili powder
- 1 tablespoon red pepper flakes
- 2 teaspoon cayenne pepper
- salt to taste

Instructions:
1) Place the pork in the crockpot and poke holes on the meat using a knife.
2) Add the rest of the ingredients in the crockpot.
3) Close the lid and set the cooking temperature to 10 hours.
4) Garnish with avocado slices.

Nutrition information: Calories per serving: 267; Carbohydrates: 10.41g; Protein: 32.17g; Fat: 11g; Sugar: 3.66g; Sodium: 551mg; Fiber: 3.6g

Pulled Pork Cucumber Sliders

This pulled pork slider recipes is low carb but it is as delicious as its high carb contemporary.

Yields: 2
Preparation Time: 10 minutes
Cooking Time: 8 hours

Ingredients:
- 1 pound pork roast
- 3 cloves of garlic, minced
- 1 onion, sliced
- 2 teaspoon cumin
- 2 teaspoon chili powder
- 1 teaspoon oregano
- 1 teaspoon pepper
- 1 teaspoon paprika
- ½ teaspoon cinnamon
- ½ teaspoon cayenne pepper
- salt to taste
- juice of 1 lime
- 2 large cucumber cut lengthwise

Instructions:
1) Place all ingredients except the cucumber in the crockpot.
2) Close the lid and cook on low setting for 8 hours.
3) Once cooked, shred the meat using fork.
4) Place shredded pork in between the slices of cucumber as though making a cucumber burger.

Nutrition information: Calories per serving: 515; Carbohydrates: 15.95g; Protein: 63.54g; Fat: 21.65g; Sugar: 6.06g; Sodium: 195mg; Fiber: 4.8g

Five-Spice Crockpot Pork Ribs

Make the best pork rib dish with your crockpot using this recipe! What's more, this recipe is easy to follow.

Yields: 8
Preparation Time: 5 minutes
Cooking Time: 8 hours

Ingredients:
- 3 pounds pork ribs
- salt and pepper to taste
- 2 teaspoon Chinese five-spice powder
- 1 jalapeno, chopped
- ¾ teaspoon garlic powder
- 2 tablespoon rice vinegar
- 2 tablespoon coconut aminos
- 1 tablespoon tomato paste

Instructions:
1) Place all ingredients inside the crockpot.
2) Close the lid and set the temperature to low.
3) Cook for 8 hours.

Nutrition information: Calories per serving: 245; Carbohydrates: 1.37g; Protein: 35.62g; Fat: 9.63g; Sugar: 0.66 g; Sodium: 120mg; Fiber: 0.2g

Simple Pork Shanks Stew

This pork stew recipe is very easy to make using ingredients you can find in your kitchen. Use your crockpot to make the most tender pork shank stew you have ever tasted.

Yields: 8
Preparation Time: 15 minutes
Cooking Time: 6 hours

Ingredients:
- 1 tablespoon olive oil
- 3 pounds pork shanks
- 3 cups onion, diced
- 4 cloves of garlic, minced
- 1 tablespoon oregano leaves
- 2 tablespoon basil leaves
- 2 teaspoon thyme leaves
- 3 cups mushrooms, chopped
- 1 teaspoon salt
- 1 tablespoon lemon zest
- juice from 1 lemon
- 1 can tomatoes
- ¾ cup pork broth

Instructions:
1) Set the crockpot to high heat and add the oil.
2) Sear the pork shanks and add the onions and garlic for 5 minutes.
3) Add oregano leaves, basil and thyme.
4) Stir in the rest of the ingredients.

5) Close the lid and set to low temperature.
6) Cook for 6 hours.

Nutrition information: Calories per serving: 251; Carbohydrates: 7.21g; Protein: 38.77g; Fat: 6.97g; Sugar: 3.37g; Sodium: 475mg; Fiber: 1.7g

Creamy Coconut Curry Pork

This creamy pork dish has a very exotic taste. Make it with ease using your crockpot.

Yields: 8
Preparation Time: 12 hours
Cooking Time: 5 hours

Ingredients:
- 2 pounds pork stew meat
- 1 ½ tablespoon curry powder
- 1 teaspoon turmeric
- 1 tablespoon ground cumin
- salt to taste
- 2 onions, chopped
- 4 cloves of garlic, minced
- 2 tablespoons ginger, grated
- 1 cup tomatoes
- 2 cups bone broth
- 1 cup coconut milk

Instructions:
1) Place pork in the bowl and add the curry powder, turmeric, ground cumin, and season with salt. Let it marinate overnight.
2) In the morning, place the marinated meat in the crockpot and add onions, garlic, ginger, and tomatoes.
3) Pour in bone broth.
4) Cook on low temperature for 5 hours.

5) Two hours before the crockpot is done, add the coconut milk. Give a stir and cover the lid

Nutrition information: Calories per serving: 337; Carbohydrates: 6.96g; Protein: 29.83g; Fat: 21.09g; Sugar: 2.76g; Sodium: 85mg; Fiber: 2.2g

Balsamic Pork Tenderloin

This recipe is easy to prepare and it will not take you five minutes to prepare everything. Just dump everything and let your crockpot do the cooking.

Yields: 8
Preparation Time: 6 minutes
Cooking Time: 6 hours

Ingredients:
- 1 tablespoon olive oil
- 4 cloves of garlic, minced
- 2 pounds pork tenderloin
- ½ cup balsamic vinegar
- 1 tablespoon Worcestershire sauce
- 2 tablespoon coconut aminos
- ½ teaspoon salt
- ½ teaspoon red pepper flakes

Instructions:
1) Drizzle oil at the bottom of the crockpot and add the garlic.
2) Add the pork tenderloin.
3) Pour in the rest of the ingredients.
4) Close the lid and cook on low temperature for 6 hours or 4 hours on high.

Nutrition information: Calories per serving: 188; Carbohydrates: 1.3g; Protein: 30.3g; Fat: 5.8g; Sugar: 0.6g; Sodium: 455mg; Fiber: 0g

Pork Medallions in Mushroom Sauce

Make this easy pork medallion recipe and make it more interesting with the mushroom sauce.

Yields: 4
Preparation Time: 15 minutes
Cooking Time: 6 hours and 8 minutes

Ingredients:
- 1 pound pork tenderloin
- ½ teaspoon salt
- ½ teaspoon black pepper
- 2 tablespoons butter
- 1 cup baby Bella mushrooms, sliced
- 1 cup chicken stock
- 1 tablespoon sage, chopped
- 1 teaspoon thyme, chopped

Instructions:
1) Sprinkle salt and pepper on pork tenderloin. Set aside.
2) Set the crockpot on high heat and melt the butter. Add the pork tenderloin and cook for 4 minutes on each side.
3) Add the mushrooms, chicken stock, sage, and thyme.
4) Close the lid and allow to cook on low for 6 hours.

Nutrition information: Calories per serving: 243; Carbohydrates: 5g; Protein: 34.1g; Fat:10.1g; Sugar: 1.3g; Sodium: 565mg; Fiber: 1g

Pork Chops with Creamy Herbed Sauce

Tired of eating fried pork chops? Then you can turn your ordinary pork chop into this creamy dish.

Yields: 6
Preparation Time: 15 minutes
Cooking Time: 8 hours

Ingredients:
- 2 pounds pork loin chops
- ½ teaspoon salt
- 1/8 teaspoon pepper
- 1 teaspoon thyme
- ½ teaspoon dried mustard powder
- 1 tablespoon olive oil
- ½ onion, diced
- 3 cloves garlic, minced
- 1 ½ cups chicken broth
- ¾ cup heavy cream
- 1 teaspoon parsley

Instructions:
1) Sprinkle pork chops with salt, pepper, thyme, and mustard powder. Set aside.
2) Set the crockpot to high heat and heat oil.
3) Sauté the onion and garlic.
4) Place the pork chops and sear for 4 minutes on each side.
5) Add the chicken broth.
6) Close the lid and set to low temperature.
7) Cook for 8 hours on low or 4 hours on high.

8) An hour before the dish is done, add the heavy cream.
9) Garnish with parsley once done.

Nutrition information: Calories per serving: 398; Carbohydrates: 2.21g; Protein: 39.67g; Fat: 24.69g; Sugar:1.15g; Sodium: 519mg; Fiber: 0.2g

Jerk BBQ Pork Ribs

Who says you only need a grill to make BBQ ribs? Make your own version of BBQ ribs in your crockpot using this recipe.

Yields: 6
Preparation Time: 8 hours
Cooking Time: 10 hours

Ingredients:
- 1 rack pork ribs
- 1 cup jerk seasoning
- ¼ cup water
- ¼ cup tamari
- 2 tablespoons ginger, grated
- 2 tablespoon orange zest
- ¼ cup white vinegar
- 1 tablespoon Worcestershire sauce
- 1 tablespoon Dijon mustard

Instructions:
1) Place all ingredients in a bowl and marinate for at least 8 hours.
2) Once marinated, place all ingredients in the crockpot.
3) Cook on low for 8 to 10 hours.

Nutrition information: Calories per serving: 320; Carbohydrates: 3g; Protein: 34g; Fat: 20g; Sugar: 0.2g; Sodium: 239mg; Fiber: 0.4 g

Buffalo Pork Chops

If you love buffalo sauce, then this pork recipe is great for you. This recipe is great for BBQ parties and just anytime you feel like eating one.

Yields: 8
Preparation Time: 10 minutes
Cooking Time: 6

Ingredients:
- 2 pounds boneless pork chops
- salt and pepper to taste
- 2 tablespoon olive oil
- 2 tablespoons butter
- 3 tablespoon commercial BBQ sauce
- ¼ cup water
- 1 cup mozzarella cheese, shredded

Instructions:
1) Season the pork chops with salt and pepper.
2) Set the crockpot to high heat and heat the olive oil and butter. Add the pork chops and cook for 3 minutes on each side.
3) Stir in the commercial BBQ sauce and water.
4) Add mozzarella cheese on top.
5) Cook on low for 6 hours.

Nutrition information: Calories per serving: 316; Carbohydrates: 1.48g; Protein: 33.77g; Fat: 18.82g; Sugar: 0.76g; Sodium: 238mg; Fiber: 0.5g

Chapter 6: Seafood Keto Crockpot Recipes

Spicy Shrimp Fra Diavolo

This spicy shrimp recipe is Italian in origin and it is popular for its spicy sauce.

Yields: 2
Preparation Time: 10 minutes
Cooking Time: 3 hours

Ingredients:
- 1 teaspoon olive oil
- 1 onion, diced
- 5 cloves of garlic, minced
- 1 teaspoon red pepper flakes
- 1 can fire roasted tomatoes
- ½ teaspoon black pepper
- salt to taste
- ¼ pound shrimp, shelled and deveined
- 1 tablespoon Italian parsley

Instructions:
1) Set the crockpot to high heat and heat the oil
2) Sauté the onion and garlic for 2 minutes.
3) Add the pepper flakes and tomatoes.
4) Season with black pepper and salt.
5) Add the shrimps.
6) Adjust the heat setting to low and cook for 2 or 3 hours.

7) Garnish with parsley.

Nutrition information: Calories per serving: 134; Carbohydrates: 3.41 g; Protein: 13.99g; Fat: 3.44 g; Sugar: 1.5g; Sodium: 609mg; Fiber: 0.4g

Savory and Spicy Garlicky Shrimp

This savory shrimp recipe is easy to make. Put all ingredients in the crockpot and you are good to go.

Yields: 8
Preparation Time: 5 minutes
Cooking Time: 10 minutes

Ingredients:
- 1 tablespoon olive oil
- 6 cloves garlic, sliced thinly
- 1 teaspoon smoked paprika
- ¼ teaspoon red pepper flakes
- 1 teaspoon salt
- ¼ teaspoon black pepper
- 2 pounds shrimp, peeled and deveined

Instructions:
1) Mix the oil, garlic, paprika, and red pepper flakes. Season with salt and pepper.
2) Add the shrimps and stir to coat evenly.
3) Cook on high for 10 minutes.

Nutrition information: Calories per serving: 133; Carbohydrates: 1.09g; Protein: 23.38g; Fat: 3.28g; Sugar: 0.12g; Sodium: 1278mg; Fiber: 0.2g

Shrimp Scampi with Spaghetti Squash

Make a healthy shrimp scampi recipe made even healthier with spaghetti squash.

Yields: 4
Preparation Time: 10 minutes
Cooking Time: 2 hours and 20 minutes

Ingredients:
- 1 cup broth
- 2 teaspoon lemon-garlic seasoning
- 1 onion, chopped
- 1 tablespoon butter
- 3 pounds spaghetti squash, cut lengthwise and seeds removed
- ¾-pounds shrimp, shelled and deveined

Instructions:
1) Pour broth in the slow cooker and add the lemon-garlic seasoning, onion and butter.
2) Place the spaghetti squash inside the slow cooker and cook on high for 2 hours until soft.
3) Add the shrimps and cook for 20 more minutes on high.

Nutrition information: Calories per serving: 239; Carbohydrates: 16.79g; Protein: 21.19g; Fat: 6.28g; Sugar: 6.63g; Sodium: 1016mg; Fiber: 5.6g

Tuna and White Beans

This recipe is a healthier version of pork and beans because it is made from tuna.

Yields: 4
Preparation Time: 10 minutes
Cooking Time: 5 hours and 15 minutes

Ingredients:
- 4 tablespoon olive oil
- 1 clove of garlic, minced
- 6 cups water
- 1 pound white beans, soaked overnight and drained
- 2 cups chopped tomatoes
- 3 cans white tuna, drained and flaked
- 2 sprigs of basil
- salt and pepper to taste

Instructions:
1) Set the crockpot to high heat and add oil.
2) Sauté the garlic for 2 minutes and add water.
3) Stir in the beans. Close the lid and cook on high for 5 hours.
4) Add in the tomatoes, tuna and basil.
5) Season with salt and pepper to taste.
6) Continue cooking on high for 15 minutes.

Nutrition information: Calories per serving: 764; Carbohydrates: 12.05g; Protein: 62.84g; Fat: 25.43g; Sugar:4 g; Sodium: 559mg; Fiber: 6.03g

Crockpot Swordfish Steaks

Make healthy steaks with this seafood recipe. Making it is as easy as 1-2-3.

Yields: 6
Preparation Time: 10 minutes
Cooking Time: 2 hours

Ingredients:
- 6 swordfish steaks
- ½ cup olive oil
- ¼ cup lemon juice
- ½ teaspoon Worcestershire sauce
- ¼ teaspoon black pepper
- 1 teaspoon cayenne pepper powder
- ¼ teaspoon paprika

Instructions:
1) Place the swordfish steaks in the crockpot.
2) Pour the other ingredients over the swordfish steaks.
3) Close the lid and cook on high for 2 hours.

Nutrition information: Calories per serving: 659; Carbohydrates: 1.63g; Protein: 46.59g; Fat: 50.78g; Sugar: 0.7g; Sodium: 113mg; Fiber: 0.2g

Rustic Fish and Tomatoes

Prepare this rustic dish of fish and tomatoes using your crockpot. This simple dish is not only simple but also delicious.

Yields: 4
Preparation Time: 10 minutes
Cooking Time: 3 hours

Ingredients:
- 1 pound cod fillet,
- 3 cloves of garlic, minced
- 1 onion, sliced
- 1 bell pepper, sliced
- 1 tablespoon rosemary
- 1 can diced tomatoes
- ¼ teaspoon red pepper flakes
- ¼ cup broth
- salt and pepper to taste

Instructions:
1) Place all ingredients in the crockpot and stir to mix well.
2) Cook on low for 3 hours or high for 30 minutes.

Nutrition information: Calories per serving:103; Carbohydrates: 5.3g; Protein: 18.68g; Fat: 0.76g; Sugar: 2.63g; Sodium: 449mg; Fiber: 1.4g

Sweet and Sour Shrimp

Make this shrimp and sour shrimp recipe with your crockpot using simple ingredients you can find in your pantry.

Yields: 3
Preparation Time: 10 minutes
Cooking Time: 5 hours

Ingredients:
- 1 package Chinese pea pods, cleaned and trimmed
- 1 can pineapple tidbits
- ½ teaspoon ginger, ground
- ½ pounds shrimps, shelled and deveined
- 1 cup chicken broth
- ½ cup pineapple juice
- 2 tablespoon apple cider vinegar
- salt to taste

Instructions:
1) Put the peas in the bottom of the crockpot.
2) Add the pineapple tidbits and ginger.
3) Place the shrimps on top.
4) Add the chicken broth
5) pineapple juice and apple cider vinegar.
6) Season with salt.
7) Cook on low for 5 hours.

Nutrition information: Calories per serving: 236; Carbohydrates: 3.5 g; Protein: 17.12 g; Fat: 1.33 g; Sugar: 1.5g; Sodium: 970 mg; Fiber:0.6g

Lazyman's Seafood Stew

This seafood stew is perfect for anyone who wants to eat a simple yet delicious meal.

Yields: 6
Preparation Time: 10 minutes
Cooking Time: 3 hours

Ingredients:
- 1 pound large shrimp
- 1 pound scallops
- 1 can crushed tomatoes
- 4 cloves of garlic, minced
- 1 tablespoon tomato paste
- 4 cups vegetable broth
- 1 teaspoon dried oregano
- ½ cup onion, chopped
- ½ teaspoon celery salt
- 1 teaspoon dried thyme
- 1/8 teaspoon cayenne pepper
- ¼ teaspoon red pepper flakes
- 2 teaspoons salt
- 2 teaspoons pepper

Instructions:
1) Put all ingredients in the crockpot and stir to combine.
2) Close the lid and cook on high for 3 hours or for 30 minutes on high setting.

Nutrition information: Calories per serving: 135; Carbohydrates: 9.26g; Protein: 20.37g; Fat: 1.29g; Sugar: 3.76g; Sodium: 1906mg; Fiber:1.3g

Halibut Vinaigrette

This halibut dish is very refreshing with its lemon vinaigrette.

Yields: 6
Preparation Time: 15 minutes
Cooking Time: 3 hours

Ingredients:
- 2 tablespoon fresh lime juice
- 1 tablespoon fresh thyme
- ½ teaspoon crushed red pepper
- salt and pepper to taste
- 4 fillets of halibut fish
- 1 bunch kale, torn
- 1 cup water
- 1 shallot, sliced

Instructions:
1) Mix together lime juice, thyme, red pepper, salt, and pepper.
2) Sprinkle the spices on the halibut fillet.
3) Place the kale in the crockpot and place the halibut fillet at the bottom.
4) Pour in water and sprinkle shallots on top.
5) Close the lid and cook on low for 2 to 3 hours.

Nutrition information: Calories per serving: 81; Carbohydrates: 1.25g; Protein: 13.68 g; Fat: 2.12g; Sugar: 0.48g; Sodium: 323mg; Fiber:0.2 g

Crockpot Crab Legs

Crab legs are favorite during picnics. Make this dish easily with your crockpot and you will never go wrong with this recipe.

Yields: 10
Preparation Time: 10 minutes
Cooking Time: 3 hours

Ingredients:
- 5 pounds crab legs
- 1 tablespoon butter
- 1 teaspoon garlic powder
- 2 lemons, juiced
- salt and pepper to taste

Instructions:
1) Place all ingredients in the pot.
2) Fill the crockpot with ¼ water.
3) Close the lid and cook on low for 3 hours.

Nutrition information: Calories per serving: 294; Carbohydrates: 1.31g; Protein: 49.27g; Fat: 8.87g; Sugar: 0.48g; Sodium: 175 mg; Fiber: 0.1 g

Asian-Inspired Ginger Tuna Steaks

The refreshing taste of ginger adds a deep, spicy and earthy flavor to this tuna steak dish.

Yields: 8
Preparation Time: 10 minutes
Cooking Time:4 hours

Ingredients:
- 2 pounds tuna steak
- 2 tablespoon coconut aminos
- 2 tablespoon sherry wine
- ½ cup water
- 6 sprigs of onion, chopped
- 3 cloves of garlic, minced
- 1 teaspoon ginger, grated
- salt and pepper to taste

Instructions:
1) Place the tuna steak at the bottom of the crockpot.
2) Add the rest of the ingredients and give a swirl to make sure that the tuna steaks are coated with the marinade.
3) Close the lid and cook on low for 3 to 4 hours.

Nutrition information: Calories per serving: 387; Carbohydrates: 12.87g; Protein: 30.65g; Fat: 20.29g; Sugar: 12.9g; Sodium: 91mg; Fiber: 2.4g

Rustic Buttered Mussels

There are many ways to cook mussels and this recipe is one of the easiest one there is that you can try.

Yields: 6
Preparation Time: 5 minutes
Cooking Time: 3 hours

Ingredients:
- 2 pounds mussels, cleaned
- ½ cup white wine
- 2 cloves of garlic, minced
- 1 ¼ tablespoon salt
- 2 tablespoons butter

Instructions:
1) Place all ingredients in the crockpot.
2) Cook on low for 3 hours or until the mussels have opened.

Nutrition information: Calories per serving: 167; Carbohydrates: 6.13g; Protein: 18.19g; Fat: 7.23g; Sugar: 0.23g; Sodium: 1918 mg; Fiber:0g

Boiled Lobster Tails

Lobster tails are one of the most expensive ingredients that you can cook. This simple recipe results to a very delicate lobster tail dish that you will ever taste.

Yields: 4
Preparation Time: 15 minutes
Cooking Time:3 hours

Ingredients:
- 4 lobster tails
- 1 cup water
- 4 ounces of white cooking wine
- ½ stick of butter
- ½ tablespoon salt
- 2 tablespoon lemon juice
- 1 teaspoon rosemary

Instructions:
1) Place all ingredients in the crockpot.
2) Cook on low for 3 hours or until the lobsters are red.

Nutrition information: Calories per serving: 151; Carbohydrates: 0.56 g; Protein: 30.9g; Fat: 2g; Sugar: 0g; Sodium: 1522mg; Fiber: 0g

Creamy Shrimp Chowder

If you are desiring a thick and creamy seafood chowder, this can be your go-to recipe. You can also sprinkle parsley flakes before serving.

Serves: 8
Cooking Time: 4 hours
Preparation Time: 15 minutes

Ingredients:
- ½ cup butter
- 1 cup heavy whipping cream
- 32-ounce chicken broth
- 2 cups sliced mushroom
- 8-ounce cheddar cheese shredded
- 24-ounce small shrimp

Instructions:
1) Place Crockpot on high settings.
2) Pour in chicken broth and mushrooms.
3) Cover and cook for two hours.
4) Stir in butter and whipping cream mix well.
5) Cover and cook for 30 minutes.
6) Stir in cheese. Mix well until cheese is melted and incorporated.
7) Cover and cook for 30 minutes, and halfway through stir to mix.
8) If needed cook for another 30 minutes more until cheese is thoroughly melted and incorporated. Stir every 15 minutes.
9) Add shrimp, stir and cook for 30 minutes.

Nutrition information: Calories per serving: 451; Carbohydrates: 4g; Protein: 29g; Fat: 33g; Sugar: 0g; Sodium: 571mg; Fiber: 0g

Keto-Approved Clam Chowder

Traditional clam chowder is not keto-approved, but for all those clam chowder fans who are on a keto diet here is one ketogenic approved recipe that you can enjoy without the repercussions!

Serves: 8
Cooking Time: 5 hours
Preparation Time: 20 minutes

Ingredients:
- 1 teaspoon pepper
- 1 teaspoon salt
- 1 teaspoon ground thyme
- 2 cups heavy whipping cream
- 2 cups chicken broth
- 3 cans of Fancy whole baby clams with juice
- 1 cup chopped celery
- 1 cup chopped onion
- 13 slices thick cut bacon

Instructions:
1) In a skillet, crisp fry bacon and then reserve bacon grease.
2) Crumble bacon and set aside.
3) In same skillet with bacon grease, sauté onions and celery for 5 minutes or until soft.
4) Place crockpot on low settings.
5) Pour in softened veggies along with what is left of the bacon grease into Crockpot.
6) Add all remaining ingredients into Crockpot, including the crumbled bacon.

7) Cover and cook for 5 hours.

Nutrition information: Calories per serving: 427; Carbohydrates: 5g; Protein: 27g; Fat: 33g; Sugar: 0g; Sodium: 1636mg; Fiber: 0g

Chapter 7: Breakfast and Eggs Keto Crockpot Recipes

Mocha Chia Pudding

Prepare this delicious and healthy pudding recipe to jumpstart your day. This breakfast dish is a great alternative to your coffee or chocolates.

Yields: 2
Preparation Time: 5 minutes
Cooking Time: 30 minutes

Ingredients:
- 2 tablespoon herbal coffee
- 1/3 cup dry chia seeds
- 1/3 cup coconut cream
- 1 tablespoon vanilla extract
- 2 tablespoon cacao nibs
- ½ tablespoon stevia sweetener

Instructions:
1) Place all ingredients in the crockpot.
2) Mix well until well combined.
3) Cook on high for 30 minutes.
4) Serve warm.

Nutrition information: Calories per serving: 257; Carbohydrates: 2.3g; Protein: 7g; Fat: 20.5g; Sugar: 5g; Sodium: 135mg; Fiber: 11.5g

Rustic Fisherman's Eggs

This breakfast egg recipe is not your usual dish. It is a combination of fats, protein and veggies that makes this dish very nutritious.

Yields: 1
Preparation Time: 10 minutes
Cooking Time: 2 hours

Ingredients:
- 2 eggs, cage-free
- 1 can sardines in oil
- ½ cup arugula
- 1 cup artichokes, trimmed and sliced
- a pinch of salt and pepper

Instructions:
1) Place the sardines in the bottom of the crockpot.
2) Break the eggs carefully on top of the sardines.
3) Add the arugula and artichokes on top.
4) Sprinkle with salt and pepper.
5) Close the lid and cook on low for 2 hours.

Nutrition information: Calories per serving: 315; Carbohydrates: 3.5g; Protein: 28g; Fat: 21.05g; Sugar: 2g; Sodium: 115mg; Fiber: 1.5g

Easy-Peasy Breakfast Frittata

Packed with vegetables and protein, this recipe makes one satisfying breakfast!

Yields: 8
Preparation Time: 10 minutes
Cooking Time: 3 hours

Ingredients:
- 8 eggs, beaten
- 1 1/3 cup sausages, sliced
- ¾ cup spinach
- 1 ½ cup red bell pepper, diced
- ¼ cup onion, chopped
- salt and pepper to taste

Instructions:
1) Mix all ingredients in a mixing bowl.
2) Pour in the crockpot.
3) Close the lid and cook on low for 3 hours.

Nutrition information: Calories per serving: 149; Carbohydrates: 3.24g; Protein: 10.23g; Fat: 10.53g; Sugar: 1.53g; Sodium: 147mg; Fiber: 0.5 g

Sausage and Eggs Breakfast Casserole

Packed with veggies and protein, this breakfast recipe will surely brighten your day.

Yields: 8
Preparation Time: 10 minutes
Cooking Time: 5 hours

Ingredients:
- 1 broccoli head, chopped
- 1 package sausages, sliced
- 1 cup mozzarella cheese, shredded
- 10 eggs, beaten
- ¾ cup whipping cream
- 2 cloves of garlic, minced
- salt and pepper to taste

Instructions:
1) Spray cooking oil in the interior of the crockpot.
2) Place broccoli heads and half of the sausages at the bottom of the crockpot.
3) Sprinkle ½ of the cheese on top.
4) In a mixing bowl, combine eggs, whipping cream, and garlic. Season with salt and pepper to taste.
5) Pour over the egg mixture to the vegetable and sausages.
6) Sprinkle the remaining cheese.
7) Close the lid and cook on low for 5 hours or 3 hours on high.

Nutrition information: Calories per serving: 484; Carbohydrates: 5.39g; Protein: 26.13g; Fat: 38.86g; Sugar: 0g; Sodium: 858mg; Fiber: 1.18g

Eggs Poached in Spicy Tomato Sauce (Shakshouka)

An Arabic egg dish, Shakshouka is rich in protein, healthy fats, and fiber. A perfect meal to start your day!

Yields: 4
Preparation Time: 10 minutes
Cooking Time: 15 minutes

Ingredients:
- 1 tablespoon butter
- 3 cloves of garlic, minced
- 1 onion, chopped
- 1 Serrano pepper, chopped
- 1 bell pepper, chopped
- 3 tomatoes, chopped
- 1 teaspoon paprika
- 1 teaspoon cumin
- ¼ teaspoon chili powder
- ¼ teaspoon salt
- pepper to taste
- 6 eggs
- chopped cilantro for garnish

Instructions:
1) Set the crockpot to high and melt the butter.
2) Sauté garlic and onions for three minutes.
3) Stir in the Serrano peppers, bell peppers, tomatoes, paprika, cumin, and chili powder.
4) Season with salt and pepper.

5) Let it simmer for 5 minutes.
6) Gently crack the eggs on top of the sauce and close the lid.
7) Cook on high for 5 minutes.

Nutrition information: Calories per serving: 349; Carbohydrates: 11.3g; Protein: 25.47g; Fat: 22.51g; Sugar: 5.89g; Sodium: 357mg; Fiber:2.3 g

Pine Nut Breakfast Meatballs

This simple meatball recipe is very healthy and packed with a lot of proteins.

Yields: 8
Preparation Time: 20 minutes
Cooking Time: 5 hours

Ingredients:
- 2 cups crushed tomatoes
- 4 cups fresh spinach
- 1 pound of ground beef
- 2 eggs, beaten
- ½ cups pine nuts
- ½ cup onion, shredded

Instructions:
1) Place the tomatoes and spinach in the crockpot.
2) In a mixing bowl combine the ground beef, eggs, pine nuts and onions.
3) Use your hands to form meatballs.
4) Carefully place the raw meatballs on top of the spinach-tomato sauce.
5) Close the lid and cook on low for 5 hours.

Nutrition information: Calories per serving: 246; Carbohydrates: 4.02g; Protein: 18.55g; Fat: 17.49g; Sugar: 1.81g; Sodium: 78mg; Fiber: 1.2g

Breakfast Dijon Pork "Skillet"

This recipe calls for a skillet but you can easily make it with your crockpot.

Yields: 8
Preparation Time: 10 minutes
Cooking Time: 6 hours

Ingredients:
- 1 pound ground pork
- 8 ounces mushrooms, chopped
- 2 zucchinis, sliced
- ½ teaspoon pepper
- ½ teaspoon garlic powder
- ½ teaspoon salt
- ½ teaspoon basil
- 2 tablespoon Dijon mustard

Instructions:
1) Place all ingredients in a crockpot.
2) Mix everything to combine.
3) Close the lid and cook on low for 6 hours.

Nutrition information: Calories per serving: 257; Carbohydrates: 2.11g; Protein: 17.6g; Fat: 12.21g; Sugar: 0.81g; Sodium: 234mg; Fiber: 0.2g

Gluten-Free Sausage-Crusted Quiche

This is a perfect breakfast dish that can help you sustain your entire day.

Yields: 6
Preparation Time: 20 minutes
Cooking Time: 5 hours

Ingredients:
- 12 ounces pork sausages
- 5 slices of eggplants, peeled
- 10 cherry tomatoes, halved
- 6 eggs
- 2 tablespoon whipping cream
- 2 tablespoon parmesan cheese, grated
- salt and pepper to taste
- 2 tablespoons parsley, chopped

Instructions:
1) Place the sausages and eggplants at the bottom of the crockpot.
2) Add in the tomatoes.
3) In a mixing bowl, combine the eggs, whipping cream and cheese. Season with salt and pepper.
4) Pour the egg mixture over the sausages and vegetables.
5) Top with parsley.
6) Close the lid and cook on low for 5 hours.

Nutrition information: Calories per serving: 396; Carbohydrates: 3.62 g; Protein: 20.23g; Fat: 22.2g; Sugar: 1.9g; Sodium: 641mg; Fiber: 1.4g

Overnight Breakfast Casserole

Prepare this recipe before you retire so that you will have a warm breakfast the following day.

Yields: 12
Preparation Time: 10 minutes
Cooking Time: 9 hours

Ingredients:
- ½ pound ground sausages
- 1 pound bacon, chopped
- 2 cups cheddar cheese, shredded
- 1 cup mozzarella cheese, shredded
- 1 onion, diced
- 1 green pepper, diced
- 1 red pepper, diced
- 12 eggs
- ½ cup milk
- salt and pepper to taste

Instructions:
1) Layer sausages, bacon, cheese, onions and peppers in the crockpot.
2) In a mixing bowl, mix together the eggs and milk. Season with salt and pepper.
3) Pour over the vegetables.
4) Cook on low for 8 to 9 hours.

Nutrition information: Calories per serving: 302; Carbohydrates: 6.12g; Protein: 20.35g; Fat: 22.62g; Sugar: 2.27g; Sodium: 742mg; Fiber: 1.5g

Sausage Breakfast Frittata

Made from classic breakfast favorites, this frittata recipe will give you a lot of energy to jumpstart your day.

Yields: 8
Preparation Time: 10 minutes
Cooking Time: 6 hours

Ingredients:
- 10 eggs, beaten
- 1 tablespoon basil, chopped finely
- salt and pepper to taste
- 1 package sausages, sliced
- 1 zucchini, shredded
- 1 cup cherry tomatoes, halved
- 1 cup cheddar cheese

Instructions:
1) In a mixing bowl, combine eggs and basil. Season with salt and pepper to taste. Set aside.
2) Place the sausages at the bottom of the pot, add the zucchini and cherry tomatoes.
3) Pour over the egg mixture.
4) Top with cheddar cheese.
5) Close the lid and cook on low for 6 hours.

Nutrition information: Calories per serving: 174; Carbohydrates: 2.36g; Protein: 12.03g; Fat: 12.71g; Sugar: 0.2g; Sodium: 159 mg; Fiber: 1.23g

Conclusion

There are many benefits of following the ketogenic diet. The only challenge about this particular diet is that you need to prepare healthy meals. With crockpots, you will surely be able to make different types of dishes as though you are a seasoned cook. You don't need to spend a lot of time slaving your way through the kitchen to be able to create delicious and nutritious foods. Moreover, you can still lose weight without sacrificing your meals. Let this book serve as your guide on how to create delicious dishes everyday so that you will be able to enjoy the benefits of the ketogenic diet.

Printed in Poland
by Amazon Fulfillment
Poland Sp. z o.o., Wrocław